PAPAYA

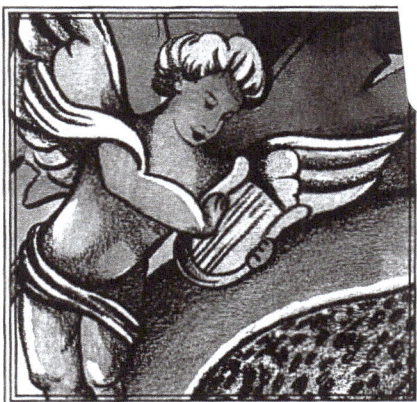

Hilary Roots

ETT IMPRINT
SYDNEY-PARIS LINK

First English edition published by ETT Imprint, Exile Bay 2023

ETT IMPRINT
PO Box R1906
Royal Exchange NSW 1225
Australia

First published in French in Noumea, New Caledonia 1996.
Reprinted 2007, 2020.

Illustrations : by Pascale Taurua

First electronic edition published by ETT Imprint 2023

Copyright © Hilary Roots, 1996, 2023

ISBN 978-1-923024-48-9 (pback)
ISBN 978-1-923024-49-6 (ebook)

*A Sydney-Paris Link publication In
memory of Jean-Paul Delamotte*

Cover : Native Flowers, 1927, hand-coloured woodcut by Margaret Preston
Design by Tom Thompson

CONTENTS

PREFACE 5

INTRODUCTION 8
By Doctor Patrick Dubois

IN PRAISE OF PAPAYA
PAPAIN, A QUALITY ENZYME 10
HEALING POWERS :
PAPAYA OINTMENT 12
FOOD FOR A POPE 13
MAY SAVE A LIFE 14
NUTRITIONAL VALUE 15
A PAPAYA DIET 16

RECIPES

HINTS TO BEGIN WITH 18
LONG DRINKS 19
COCKTAILS 24
SOUPS 26
ENTRÉES 30
SALADS 39
DRESSINGS 43
SIDE DISHES 48
MAIN DISHES 56
DESSERTS 64
COFFEE COMPANY 76

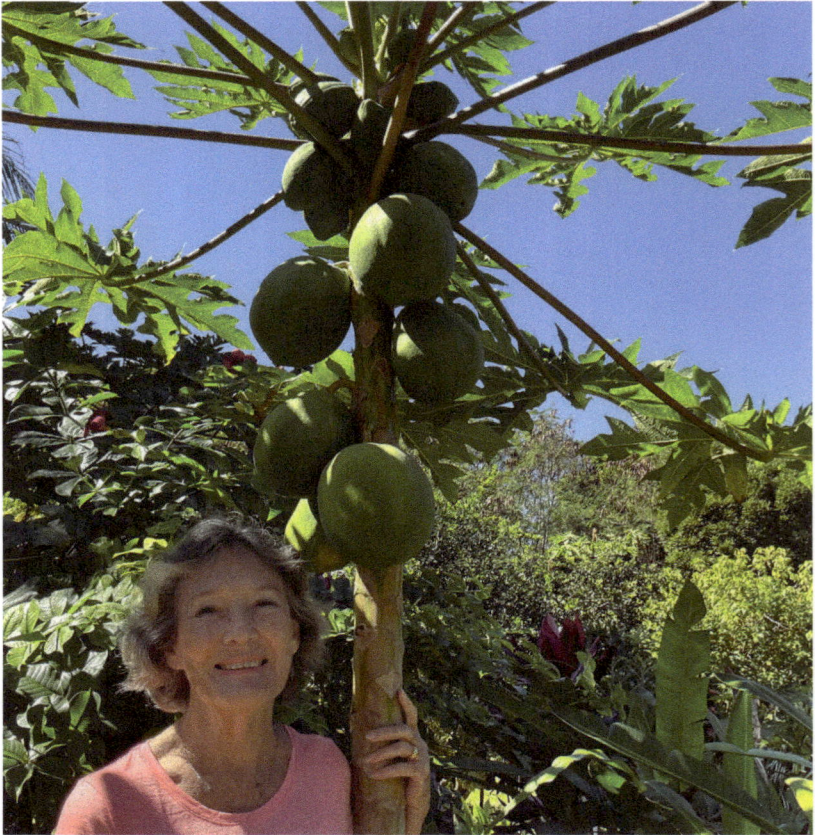

The author Hilary Roots in her garden.

PREFACE

A Caribbean friend, a cheerful, robust, creative man who loved to cook was the inspiration for this small book. Sam Bagassien was his name. His restaurant was simply Chez Sam. These pages are a tribute to him.

His venue was a little wooden cottage set amongst coconut palms and pine trees, five minutes' walk from one of the most beautiful white sand beaches in the Pacific - Kuto Bay, Isle of Pines, New Caledonia.

Chez Sam had no display sign, nor any electricity, but from the gas-lit kitchen and wood stove, emanated such enticing smells, they seemed to hang in the surrounding tropical bush, luring would-be diners. Cooking, to Sam, was a pleasure, and such pleasure was catching. His dishes had a sparkle in them, just as his kitchen echoed with laughter and his ebony body rippled harmoniously whenever he danced to Caribbean rhythms.

Sam had another reason to be proud of his cooking – using his culinary talent, including a restaurant he'd run in Noumea, called *La Canne à Sucre,* he'd helped his sister through Medical School in Paris. There weren't too many black, women doctors in the French capital, he liked to say, and probably that still rings true.

In his recipes, Sam used the most basic and often most common tropical vegetables and fruits ... chokoes, sweet potatoes, pumpkin, and the list went on to include fennel, papayas and mangoes. But instead of just boiling them, serving them raw or even ignoring them, he created palate-flattering marvels. Much of the spirit of his cooking came from his Guadaloupean origins, while the French influence in those islands enhanced his food preparation and presentation.

Intrigued, I began visiting him. We chatted. I mostly listened, copying down his recipes, as he himself had nothing written. Eventually the idea for a small book narrowed down to the papaya because it kept revealing itself in so many new guises.

I learnt that this fruit, gathered all year, was also a vegetable. That some of the small trees with star-shaped leaves, carried female flowers, others male. That the seeds, scattered on the ground, would give rise a year later to young trees. That their fruit was rich in vitamins. That they grow in the tropical and semi-tropical belt encircling the globe.

And so I set about searching for recipes based on papaya, innovating and experimenting, sometimes with some surprising taste results. I tried to keep Sam's enthusiasm, his simplicity and fun in preparing and sharing food. Dr. Patrick Dubois helped my research and the idea for a book began taking shape.

"White sand, warm sun, French food" ... those few words in an Australian newspaper first tempted me to come to Isle of Pines back in 1975. I never intended to become a chronicler of others' eating tastes and habits, but daily contact with French people accentuates the high priority they give to *la bonne cuisine*.

Today, years after having met Sam and discovering the papaya, I hope readers will not only enjoy learning about "the fruit of the angels" and ways to use it, but will also have the pleasure of sharing and savouring new palate sensations round a friendly table.

Bon appétit!

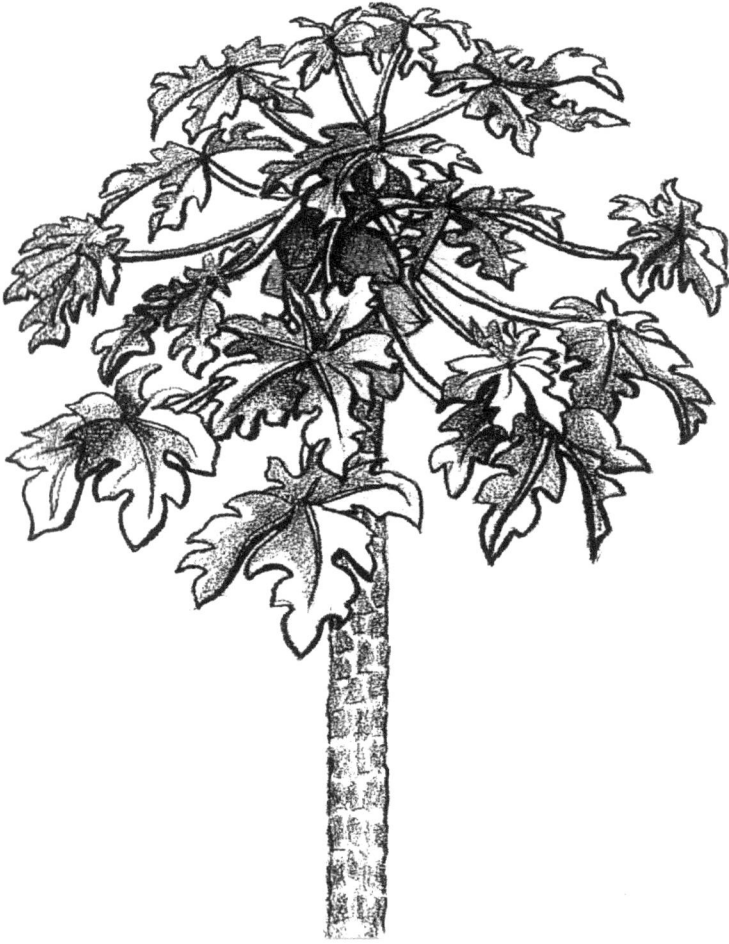

INTRODUCTION

Knowledge of the qualities of this tropical fruit/vegetable is not at all a recent discovery. The papaya caught Christopher Colombus' attention the first time he landed in the Caribbean, where he noted these healthy people lived mainly on 'a tree melon' called 'fruit of the angels'; furthermore, it could be picked all year round.

Intriguing, original, a traveller, easy to grow, generous, sometimes even a little mysterious, the papaya tree we may think we know, living so close to it every day in warm regions, is in fact complete and complex. This papaya tree, laden with fruit or exotic tassels of flowers, hides a wealth of virtues.

The papaya tree that botanists call *carica papaya* originated from Mexico, although there are claims that it really came from the Papaya district of Peru. Easily grown, it was introduced in Africa then Asia and is now found in all tropical or sub-tropical climates, including most of the Pacific.

Cultivating it is child's play - suffice to scatter a handful of seeds from a freshly-cut, ripe papaya and it will adapt to almost any soil, provided it is well drained and aerated. It likes water but not flooding nor stagnant water. It also prefers protection from strong wind. Quite extraordinarily it bears flowers and fruit all year round, as long as it's pollinated. The fruit however ripen more easily in the warmer months.

The ideal growth temperature seems to be between 22° and 26°C (72° - 80°F), as lower temperatures produce rather tasteless fruit. Frost kills the papaya tree and it can be safely said where the banana grows the papaya flourishes. Polygamous, a male plant will fertilise ten females. It can sometimes be hermaphrodite, changing sexes doesn't seem to upset it. This transexuality can be provoked by a small blow. Pierce the trunk of a male tree when it's still young with a small piece of wood and there, without cosmetic surgery or hormone treatment, you have a productive tree! It lives three to five years, and sometimes longer.

The papaya is a big, round or oval, smooth-skinned fruit, weighing from one to three kilos. When ripe, the skin (which is inedible) is yellow or orange. On cutting it open you find a cavity filled with black seeds that have a peppery taste. The juicy, slightly sweet flesh will be yellow, orange or deep pink. A slice of fresh, ripe papaya seems to melt in the mouth, flattering the taste buds and moistening the palate with a delicate perfume. The smooth flesh is easily digested and contains few calories - in all, a gift of nature.

For normally little cost (except in countries where it's imported), this bountiful fruit can be used as a drink, an appetizer, it can accompany fish or meat, replacing a vegetable. It is excellent as a salad, delicious as a preserve and proves well as a variety of desserts.

Hilary, known as *Cléo* in New Caledonia, will introduce you to her papaya secrets, the result of a natural style of cooking mixed with a delight in discovering yet new ways of using this common, if rather little understood, tropical benefactor. Impregnated now with French influence, Cleo the 'alchemist' is still looking for a recipe for papaya cheese!

P.D.

PAPAIN
A QUALITY ENZYME

Papain is a milky sap found in the leaves, stalks, bark and, in lesser amounts, in the flesh of the papaya fruit. It acts as an enzyme, in dissolving and digesting albumin-type proteins (remember the 'glutton enzymes' of the 1970s). It can be obtained easily by 'bleeding' the skin of a green papaya - simply score it lengthwise, at regular intervals, with a knife.

Papain has numerous uses:

* When **meat** or **octopus** is likely to be tough, wrap it in papaya leaves for twelve hours to soften, or rub papain into the flesh. Tenderize **poultry** by replacing the innards with a piece of papaya and leave till next day.

* A tastier **tenderiser** for meat or poultry is to cover meat with a **marinade** made by mixing in a blender a ripe papaya (peeled and deseeded) and mixed herbs. Leave to macerate for twelve hours or overnight and cook as you wish, using the marinade as a sauce.

* Sooth **insect bites**, or even counteract the **venom** from poisonous bites, by rubbing with papaya sap. But be careful, **don't touch your eyes!**

* Mix four teaspoons of sap from a green papaya with the same amount of honey in a cup of warm water. Drink it as an effective **vermifuge**.

* It's possible to **wash clothes** and **take out stains** by using crushed papaya leaves.

*   **Digestion** of red and white meats, eggs and fish is aided by accompanying them with papaya.

*   For those who suffer from a **bad back**, a treatment developed in Canada in the early 80s using injections of papain, is said to produce good results for certain types of slipped discs.

*   Relief from the effects of **fish poisoning** (*ciguatera* - sometimes found in coral waters) and also **hangovers** may be had by drinking the water in which green papaya has been cooked.

HEALING POWERS
PAPAYA OINTMENT

Early in the twentieth century a Queensland medical doctor and botanist, Dr. T.P. Lucas, undertook an in-depth study of the papaya tree. This led him to declare: "The *Carica Papaya* is without doubt the most wonderful tree in the world. Its properties as agencies of life are, I believe, unparalleled. Its power of healing wounds is accelerated by its antiseptic properties".

No doubt, Dr. Lucas had isolated the qualities of papain. From what he called 'fermented papayate' he developed a translucent ointment he trade-named *Papaw Ointment*, believing 'papaw' to be logical derivative of the botanical 'papaya'. The ointment can be rubbed on the skin or swallowed in small half-teaspoon quantities, depending on the problem.

It is said to be effective for a wide range of annoying pains such as aching joints and muscles, stomach ulcers, catarrh and sinus, as well as numerous skin problems - cuts, boils, sores, open wounds, eczema, dermatitis, nappy/diaper rash, stings and bites. Cleo herself has seen good results with Dr. Lucas' ointment in aiding healing burns.

P.D.

FOOD FOR A POPE

The fact that a recent Pope included Papaya in his wellness diet, might interest some readers.

It was not on any whim that Pope Jean-Paul II ('the Polish Pope' 1978-2005) began eating the "fruit of the angels" daily, but on the recommendation of Nobel Prize winner, Professor Luc Montagnier, recognised for having discovered the Aids virus.

The French doctor (deceased early 2022), suggested the Pope eat papaya to help counteract his having Parkinson's disease. The recommendation was controversial and without proof, however, those who knew the Pope in the early years of 2000, remarked he was sprightlier for consuming the enzyme and vitamin C-rich fruit.

H.R.

MAY SAVE A LIFE

Local knowledge in Vanuatu (New Caledonia's northern neighbour) reveals the contribution a green papaya can make in an urgent situation where someone is unfortunate to be stung by a stone fish. Highly venomous stone fish can provoke severe shock with a sting from one of their 13 dorsal spines.

Vanuatais react as quickly as possible by heating a green papaya over a fire or in an oven. Once hot, they carefully handle the fruit, cut it in half, seeds and all, and apply the hot, cavity side to the wound, keeping it in place for about an hour, or until the shock and pain have subsided.

Poisonous stings from stone fish or other sea creatures contain protein and need a temperature of 60° or more to dilute them. Of course care needs to be taken not to burn the patient. The effectiveness of the hot papaya held in place over the sting, is not attributed to the papaya itself but to its preserving heat over the long period.

H.R.

NUTRITIONAL VALUE

Ripe papaya is rich in Vitamin A - indispensable for good growth and vision, and in Vitamin C - needed for tissue growth, iron absorption and basic metabolism. With a dash of lime or lemon juice, a slice of ripe papaya is excellent for sore throats.

One hundred grams (3½ ounces) of papaya yield :
- 45 glucide calories (sugar)
- 4 protide calories (protein)
- 1 lipide calorie (fat)
- water.

Baby will appreciate a very small quantity (1 or 2 teaspoons per day) of ripe papaya blended into a juice (without sugar) from three months onward. From the fourth month, babies can take ripe papaya crushed into a purée (again in small quantities). Papaya is good for children's physical growth and being rich in Vitamin C makes it a suitable basic part of an adult's daily intake. For sick people, it's an ideal aid to convalescence.

A PAPAYA DIET

Thinking about a diet, then consider papaya!

Take for example, two kilos (4½ lbs) of papaya, enhanced by the addition of lime or lemon juice, accompanied by low-fat milk products (unsweetened, plain yoghurt for example), lettuce and a hard-boiled egg or a small steak each day.

You can lose three to four kilos (6 – 9 pounds) in a week this way! Try and you'll see. It could be the solution to figure worries you've been looking for, especially if you have a sedentary activity.

Indeed, whether you're svelte or not so svelte, young or not so young, well or not so well, the Pacific without papayas, would be like an evening without a sunset.

Doctor Patrick Dubois
Specialist in Preventive and Social Medicine
Noumea / Paris.

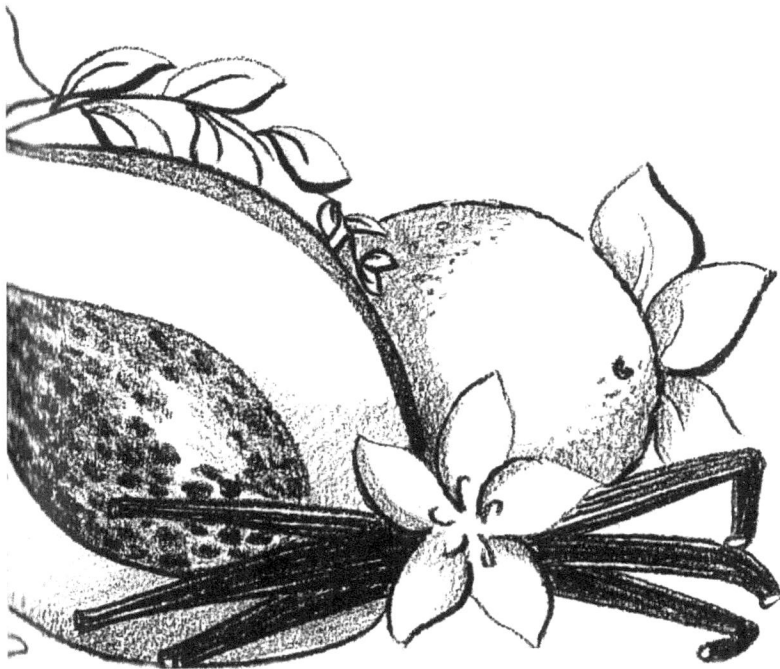

HINTS TO BEGIN WITH

1 small papaya	=	400-500 grams / approx. 1 pound
1 medium papaya	=	approx. 1 kilo / 2 - 2½ pounds
1 large papaya	=	1,5 - 2 kilos / 3½ - 4½ pounds

For each green papaya, in all recipes (unless keeping the skin is specifically mentioned) prepare as follows: make five or six incisions from top to tail in the skin to bleed the milky sap, which is bitter. Then rinse the fruit under running water, cut off the bottom of the fruit to stand it easily on a chopping board, peel off the green skin with a kitchen knife and scrape out the seeds with a spoon.

Abbreviations commonly used :

tsp	=	teaspoon	oz	=	ounce(s)
tbsp	=	tablespoon	lb	=	pound(s)
min	=	minute(s)	g	=	gram(s)
doz	=	dozen	kg	=	kilogram(s)
hr	=	hour(s)	lit	=	litre

Note: 1 tbsp = approx. 15 grams

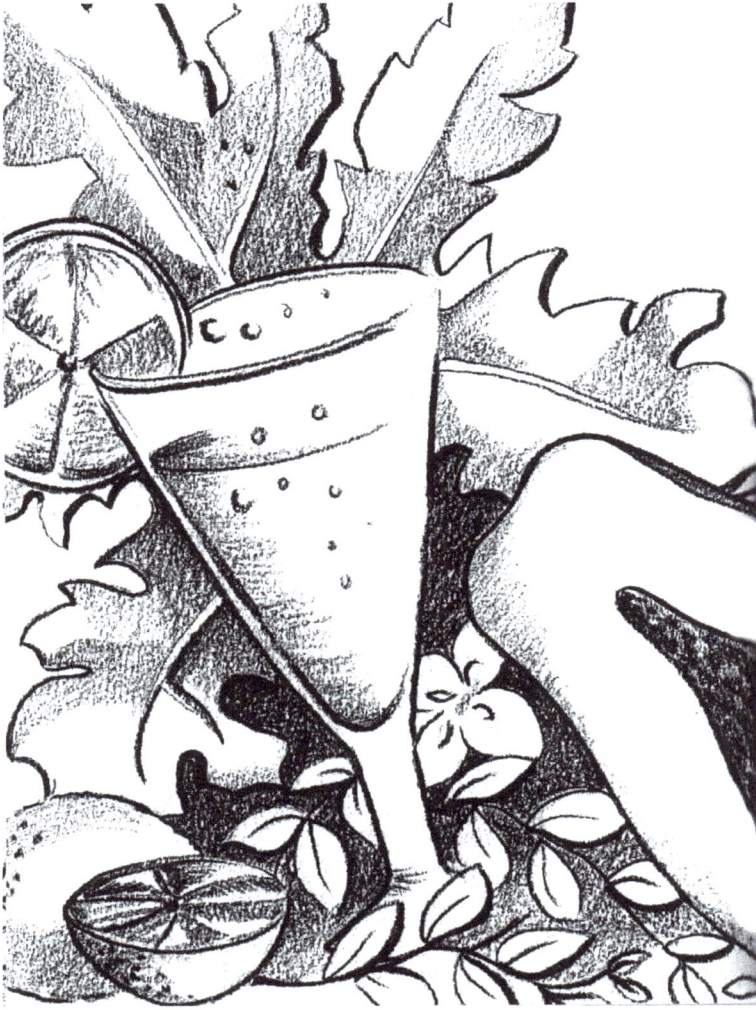

LONG DRINKS

ORANGE ICE

(for 6 pers.)

1 medium, ripe papaya
2 tbsp sugar
juice of 1 lime or lemon
2 cups cold water
2 cups orange juice
ice cubes

- Peel, deseed papaya.
- Blend to a purée with sugar & lime juice.
- Mix well with water & orange juice.
- Pour over ice; decorate glasses with a thin slice of orange.

PAPAYA LASSI

(for 4 pers.)

1 small ripe papaya
juice of 2 or 3 limes/lemons
2 pots (= 1 cup) natural, unsweetened yoghurt
ice

- Peel, deseed papaya.
- Blend all till smooth.
- Serve well chilled.

* This drink, of Indian origin, is most refreshing. Sugar or a pinch of salt can be added according to taste.

PAPAYA SHAKE

(for 6 pers.)	(for one pers.)
1 ripe papaya	1 slice ripe papaya
3 glasses milk	½ glass milk
juice of 1 lime/lemon	squeeze of lime/lemon juice

- Peel, deseed papaya.
- Blend all to a creamy beverage.
- Serve chilled.
  * For a more elegant drink, serve with a scoop of vanilla
    ice-cream and a slice of lime or lemon on edge of glass.

PICK-ME-UP

(after a food intoxication) for 1 pers.

slice of ripe papaya, peeled, deseeded
juice of ½ or 1 lime
small slice of ginger, peeled & chopped – about 1 tsp.
a little water
1 tsp honey, if wished

- Blend all in a mixer.

PINK REFERESHER

(for 4 pers.)

1 small ripe papaya
same quantity of ripe watermelon
juice of 2 limes or lemons
1 cup water
ice

- Blend peeled, de-seeded fruit with lime juice and water.
- Serve over ice.
    * This drink is not at all sweet, but refreshing and good for slimming.

REFRESCO

(for 4 -6 pers.)

1 medium, ripe papaya (peeled, deseeded)
2 tbsp sugar
1 cup milk
several drops of vanilla essence
¼ cup lime juice or ½ cup lemon juice
grated zest of lime/lemon
cinnamon or nutmeg for sprinkling
1 cup crushed ice

- Blend all except spices and ice.
- Serve over ice and sprinkle with spice.

REVITALISER

(for 4-6 pers.)

¼ litre (1 cup) ripe papaya pulp
¼ litre (1 cup) ripe mango pulp
¼ litre (1 cup) lime/lemon juice
liquid honey

- Peel papaya & mango and de-seed.
- Blend fruit & juice till smooth.
- Sweeten with honey ; blend again.
- Chill before serving.

    * In the Caribbean this revitaliser is used as an antidote to over-eating, especially during the festive season.

SMOOTHY

(for 2 pers.)

½ small ripe papaya (peeled, de-seeded)
½ cup natural, unsweetened yoghurt
½ cup milk
3 tsp honey

- Blend all till creamy smooth.
    For a tastier, richer version add a small ripe banana and a scoop of vanilla ice-cream.

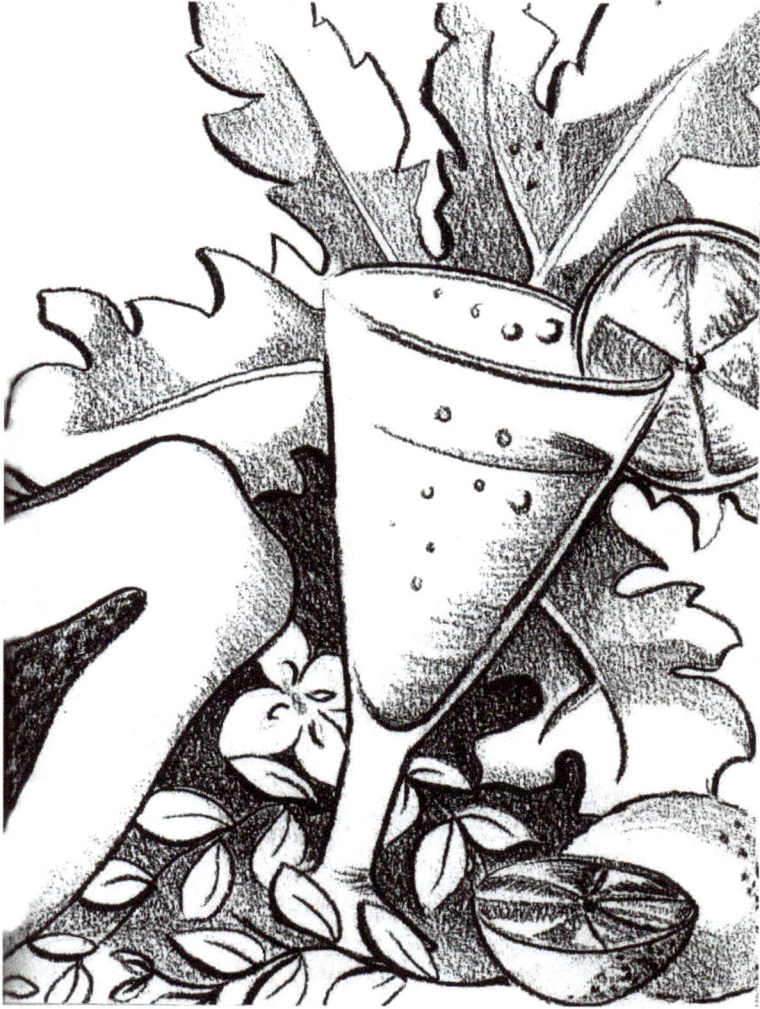

COCKTAILS

SUNSET

(for 8 pers.)

1 small ripe papaya
2 cups cold water
2 cups orange juice
2 liqueur glasses (1/2 cup) gin
juice 1 lime/lemon
1 tbsp sugar-cane syrup or sugar
ice cubes

- Peel, de-seed and chop up papaya.
- Put all ingredients, except ice, in blender, mix till smooth.
- Serve over ice cubes in flute glasses.
- Decorate with thin slice of orange or lime or lemon.

MOONBEAM

(for 6-8 pers.)

1 small ripe papaya, preferably pink
2 glasses water
1 liqueur glass (1/4 cup) rum
1 tbsp sugar-cane syrup or sugar
juice 1 lime/lemon
ice cubes
several fresh sprigs of mint

- Peel, de-seed and chop up papaya.
- Put all ingredients, except ice, in blender and mix till smooth.
- Serve over ice cubes in flute glasses.
- Decorate with a sprig of mint or slice of lime or lemon.

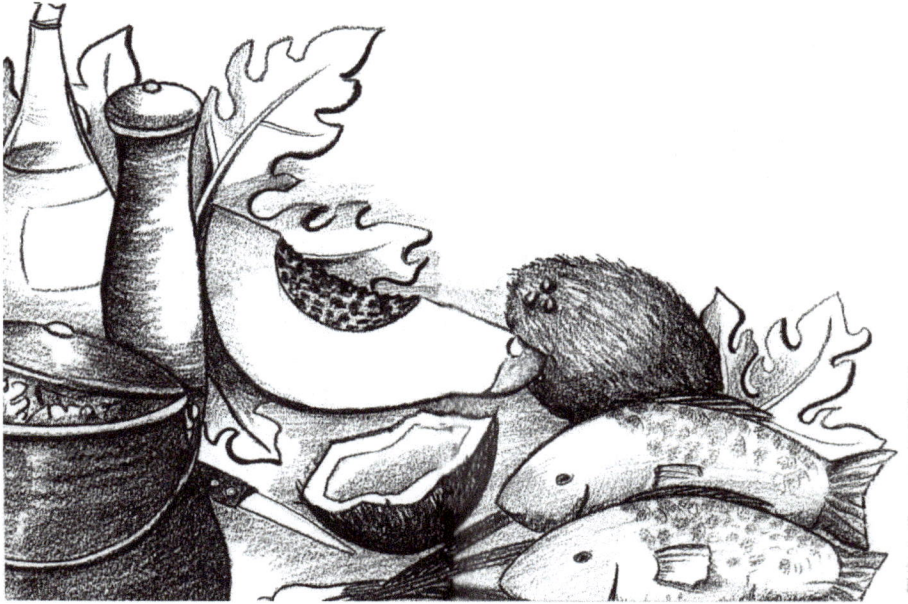

SOUPS

CHILLED SPARKLE

Consommé Glacé

(for 4-5 persons)

1 cup light syrup stock (see below)

1 medium papaya - not over-ripe

¼ bottle dry champagne

mint leaves for decoration

Make syrup stock - the rest of which can be used later to make fresh lime or lemon juice or papaya and lime juice:

1) Dissolve 175g (6oz) white sugar in ½ litre (2 cups) of water.

2) Bring to boil for one minute.

3) Remove from heat and add another ½ litre (2 cups) of water.

4) Leave to cool.

- To prepare the consommé:
- Peel and de-seed the papaya and blend in a mixer.
- Add 1 cup of the light syrup stock, then the champagne.
- Gently blend all.
- Pour into a soup tureen or individual bowls and chill.
- Garnish with mint leaves.

Recipe courtesy of the Regent Hotel, Auckland, New Zealand.

TROPICAL TRINITY

(for 4 persons)

1 medium green papaya
4 cups water
fillets of fish - approx. 1 kg (2-2½ lb)
1 onion, chopped
1 tbsp soya sauce or 1 tsp salt
pepper
1 tsp coriander seeds crushed in a garlic press
2 kaffir lime leaves (optional)
1 cup coconut milk or ½ tin (200 ml / ¾ cup) coconut cream
parsley, chopped or garlic chives, chopped

- Fillet fish, dice into bite-size pieces; keep cool.
- Peel and de-seed green papaya and grate coarsely.
- Bring water to boil, add papaya, onion, soya sauce or salt, crushed
  coriander seeds and kaffir lime leaves, if using, and cook till tender -
  approx 10 minutes.
- Add fish pieces; cook about 3 minutes.
- Lower heat. Add coconut milk or cream, pepper, parsley or garlic chives
  - mix gently - don't boil.
- Serve if wished with more parsley on top.

* To prepare coconut milk: grate flesh of 1 ripe, brown coconut ;
squeeze in a cloth to wring out milk; add enough water to make up
quantity needed.

ERIN TOUGH

(for 4-6 persons)

1 medium green papaya
3 or 4 medium potatoes
1 medium onion, chopped
2 cloves garlic, chopped
1 tbsp cooking oil
1 tbsp butter
1 glass white wine
1½ litres (1½ quarts) chicken stock
– preferably fresh, or with cube
salt, pepper
1 tsp coriander seeds, crushed in a garlic press
bunch fresh parsley and thyme

- Prepare then peel papaya and potatoes, cube.
- Heat oil and butter in a pressure cooker or other heavy pot, cook onion till transparent, add garlic.
- Add papaya and potatoes, stirring on low heat for a few minutes.
- Deglaze with white wine.
- Add stock, salt, pepper, crushed coriander seeds, parsley and thyme.
- Cook 15 minutes if using pressure cooker or slowly for 1 hour otherwise. Check if needs more water and heat through
- Remove parsley and thyme stalks; mix to a creamy consistency.
- Serve with chopped, fresh parsley on top.

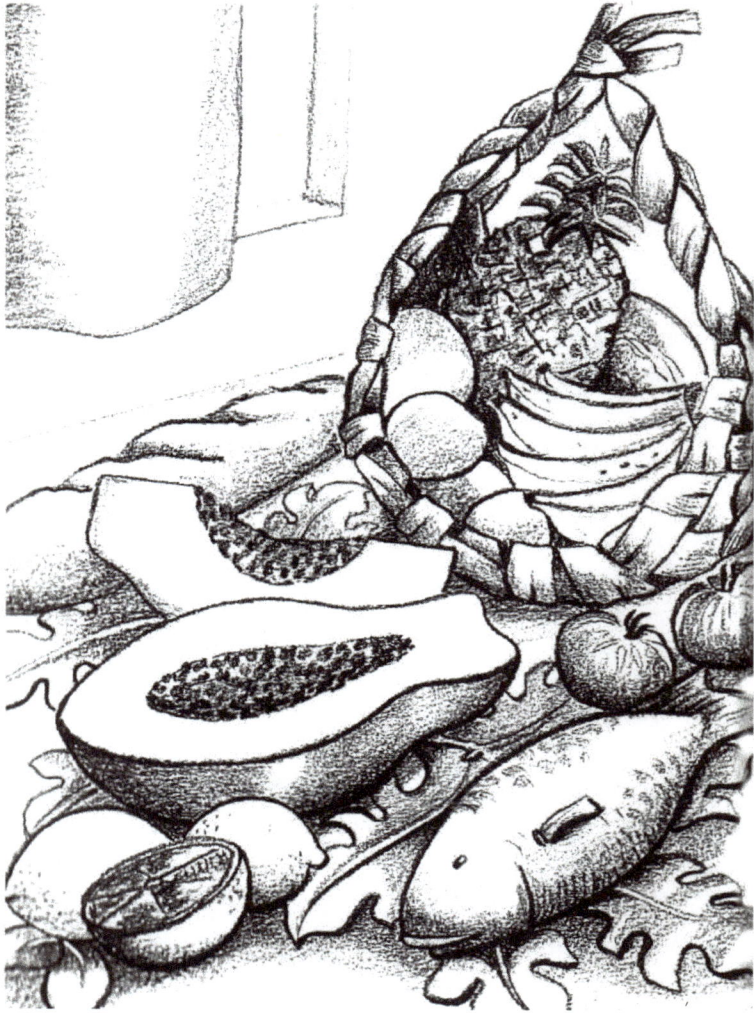

ENTRÉES
or FIRST COURSES

EASY AS CHEESE

GRATIN

(for 8 pers.)

2 kg (4½ lb) green papaya
3 eggs
salt, pepper
60g (2 oz) butter
100g (3½ oz) grated tasty cheese

- Prepare the papaya, cut into cubes, cook in salted, boiling water till soft; drain.
- In a large bowl, slightly beat eggs; salt and pepper well.
- Add papaya and butter to the eggs.
- Put mixture in a buttered gratin dish, sprinkle with grated cheese; cook in moderate oven (375º) or under grill for 10-15 minutes, till golden.

HINT OF FIJI

(for 4 pers.)

1 medium green papaya
2 medium onions, finely chopped
2 cloves garlic, cooking oil
2 tsp curry powder
salt, pepper
½ litre (2 cups) water
fresh coriander or parsley - finely chopped with 1 clove garlic

- Prepare papaya, cut into large cubes; cook in boiling, salted water till soft; drain.
- Gently brown chopped onions and garlic in oil, stir in curry powder, gently cook then add water, papaya, salt and pepper.
- Cook slowly for 20 minutes; Transfer to hot dish.
- Serve sprinkled with coriander/garlic or parsley/garlic mix.

PIED PAPAYA
(for 6-8 pers.)

1 medium (1 kg – 2-2½ lb) green papaya
2 medium onions, chopped
knob of butter
20 cl (¾ cup) thick fresh cream
1 dsp (2 tsp) French mustard
grated nutmeg
salt, pepper
puff pastry for topping
1 beaten egg yolk or milk for topping

- Prepare green papaya and grate finely.
- Sweat onions and papaya in pan in butter.
- Stir in fresh cream, mustard; season well, adding nutmeg.
- Pre-heat oven to moderately hot.
- Roll out pastry to ½ cm (¼ inch) thick and about 3 cm (an inch) larger than top of buttered pie dish. Cut 2 strips 1½ cm (½ inch) wide from pastry, stretch around lips of dish, press in place, moisten with a little cold water.
- Pour papaya mixture into pie dish.
- Drape pastry over rolling pin and unfold over dish. With a fork, crimp pastry edges together; trim with a sharp knife.
- Make several incisions in pastry, brush with beaten egg yolk or milk.
- Bake 35-40 mins. or till pastry is golden.

AIR BUBBLES

Soufflé

(for 6-8 pers.)

1 medium green papaya to make approx.
500g (1 lb) purée
50g (1½ oz) butter
3 tbsp milk
salt, pepper
thyme, fresh or dried
3 egg yolks
4 egg whites (beaten stiffly with a pinch of salt)
100g (3½ oz) grated cheese

- Prepare papaya and cut into small chunks.
- Cook in boiling, salted water.
- Pre-heat oven to moderate 190ºC (375ºF).
- Mostly drain, then mash papaya, or mix in blender.
- Add to purée the butter, milk, pepper, thyme, most of the cheese and the egg yolks.
- Gently add the stiffly beaten whites.
- Pour into buttered souffle dish, sprinkle with rest of cheese and a few knobs of butter.
- Cook in oven about 25-30 minutes till golden.
- Serve immediately.

FRENCH COUNTRY

Terrine

(for 6-8 persons)

1 kg (2-2½ lb) green papaya
cooking oil and a knob of butter
2 medium onions
3 eggs
1 level tsp. cumin powder
salt, pepper
mayonnaise (for accompaniment)

- Prepare green papaya and grate finely.
- Lightly brown onions in butter and oil.
- Add papaya and cook a few minutes too; leave to cool slightly.
- Break eggs into papaya/onion mixture, add cumin, salt, pepper and stir.
- Pour into a buttered meat-loaf tin; bake bain-marie (water to within 4cm (1½ inches) of top of terrine tin) in moderate oven 30-40 minutes or till lightly browned.
- Leave to cool.
- Turn out on to a serving platter; serve lukewarm or cold, with mayonnaise. This terrine goes nicely with a green salad to make a luncheon dish.

INDIAN OCEAN
Gratin
(for 4 persons)

1 medium green papaya or 2 small ones
3 tbsp cooking oil
1 medium onion
3 cloves garlic, chopped
1 tbsp flour
1 egg, beaten
salt, pepper
breadcrumbs
grated cheese
knob of butter

- Prepare papaya, cut into small pieces; boil in salted water about 20 minutes till well soft.
- Drain, then mash.
- Heat oil, brown chopped onion, then garlic for just a moment.
- Add flour, stirring all the time, then papaya.
- Add slightly beaten egg, salt and pepper.
- Put a knob of butter in ovenproof gratin dish or individual large scallop shells; pour in mixture. Sprinkle with breadcrumbs and grated cheese.
- Bake in moderate oven or under grill 10-15 minutes, till golden.

  * Options: add chopped crabmeat, flaked cooked fish or shrimps.

PACIFIC BREEZE
Sam's Gratin

(for 4 persons)

1 kg (2-2½ lb) green papaya
stock cube (chicken or vegetable)
bechamel sauce :   50g (1½ oz) butter
                    3 tbsp flour
                    ½ litre (2 cups) warmed milk
                    pepper
                    grated nutmeg
                    several fresh basil leaves (optional)
                    salt
                    125ml (½ cup) dry white wine (optional)
                    grated cheese
                    breadcrumbs

- Prepare papaya, quarter, cook in water with stock cube till soft; drain.
- Prepare béchamel: melt butter, blend in flour then slowly add milk,
  stirring all the time over low heat to thicken. Season generously with
  nutmeg, pepper, chopped basil (if desired); taste; salt only when
  finished (as the stock cube may make the dish quite salty).
- Stir white wine into béchamel, if desired, for a lighter, more
  aromatic sauce.
- Slice cooked papaya thinly (like apples) into sauce.
- Pour into buttered oven-proof gratin dish; top with breadcrumbs
  and grated cheese.
- Bake in moderate oven 10-15 min. till golden.
      * This dish makes an excellent entrée/starter to a meal. It can
also be a luncheon dish with hard-boiled eggs, or can accompany meat
or fish. It was Sam's regular dish and the one which introduced me to
green papaya.

COOL CLASSIC

(uncooked, per person)

1 slice ripe papaya (peeled and de-seeded)
1 or 2 slices prosciutto ham
several capers
freshly ground pepper
wedge lime or lemon
port (optional)

- Decorate individual entrée plates with the above, adding a few drops of port on each slice of papaya if desired.

TANGY TOUCH

(uncooked)

1 green papaya
mayonnaise made with a large quantity of French mustard
(2½ tbsp) & juice of 1 lime or lemon, salt & pepper

- Prepare the green papaya and grate finely.
- Mix with mayonnaise and serve cooled.

GRATIN MAISON

(for 4 pers.)

1 medium green papaya
2 cloves garlic

sauce :
150 – 200g grated cheese
1 egg
50 ml dry white wine
150 ml liquid cream
salt, pepper

- Prepare papaya, slice finely, cook till soft in boiling, salted water with slightly chopped garlic. Drain.
- Preheat oven to 180° C.
- Prepare gratin sauce, mixing ingredients in a bowl.
- Pour papaya into a buttered oven dish; cover with gratin sauce.
- Cook in oven for 10-15 minutes, then under the grill for a few minutes till golden.
- This dish can make a luncheon or main dish for 2 persons.
- An alternative can be to fry some bacon bits and mix them through the sauce.

* The quantities of cheese, white wine and cream can be varied according to taste and/or availability – as long as you obtain a good consistency when preparing with a wooden spoon.

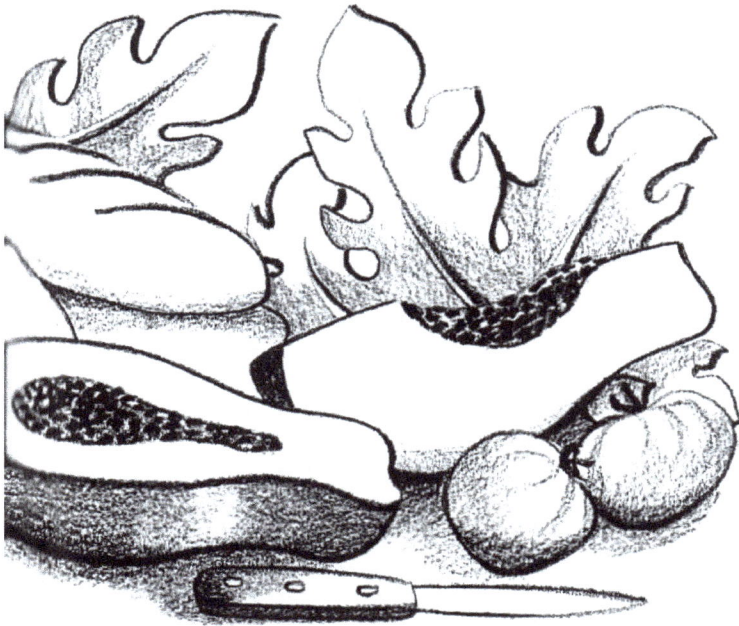

SALADS

CURRIED

(for 4-5 pers.)

1 medium firm ripe papaya
1 tsp curry powder
½ cup vinaigrette - see recipe Everyday French
lettuce leaves
1 small onion

- Mix vinaigrette into curry powder in small bowl; leave ½ hr for curry to dissolve.
- Peel, de-seed and dice papaya; coat with dressing and chill.
- Serve on lettuce leaves; decorate with onion rings.

* Goes well with cold chicken or meat.

SLICE OF RIPE

(per person)

1 slice ripe papaya - unpeeled, de-seeded
1 or 2 lettuce leaves
vinaigrette

- Arrange papaya on lettuce leaves on individual small plates.

Serve vinaigrette to accompany.

COOKED GREEN
(for 4-5 persons)

1 medium (1 kg / 2-2½lb) green papaya
parsley
2 cloves garlic
3 or 4 spring onions
vinaigrette
3 hard-boiled eggs

- Prepare papaya, quarter and cook in boiling, salted water till soft.
- Drain, cool, then slice finely, like apples.
- Finely chop herbs together; add to papaya, pour vinaigrette over and garnish with sliced hard-boiled eggs.

Variations to cooked green papaya salad :

Add 250g (½ lb) cooked, deboned fish or several anchovy fillets or a small tin of tuna or
Add 250g (½ lb) diced ham and 1 tbsp capers.

BRUSH ISLAND GREEN

(for 4-5 persons)

1 medium (1 kg / 2-2½ lb) green papaya
garlic vinaigrette (see recipe)

- Prepare papaya - i.e. 'bleed', rinse, peel and de-seed it; then grate finely (like carrots).
- Set aside in fridge (preferably an hour or two) till ready to use.
- Mix in garlic vinaigrette just before serving.

* This salad is ideal for a large group of people - simply adjust the proportions. Any quantity of vinaigrette can be made, provided you respect the basic rule of 1/3rd vinegar, 2/3rds oil.

* In the days when we took visitors by boat to picnic on heavenly Brush Island, this was part of the staple menu we served to accompany barbequed fish or lobster. For most people it was a surprising and delectable discovery.

Variations to above green papaya salad:

Instead of garlic vinaigrette, season with :
juice of 2 limes/lemons, 4 tbsp olive oil, salt & pepper
or
4 tbsp mayonnaise, salt & pepper and decorate with hard-boiled eggs.
or
2-3 tbsp soya sauce, a few drops sesame oil, a few drops tabasco, 2 crushed cloves garlic.

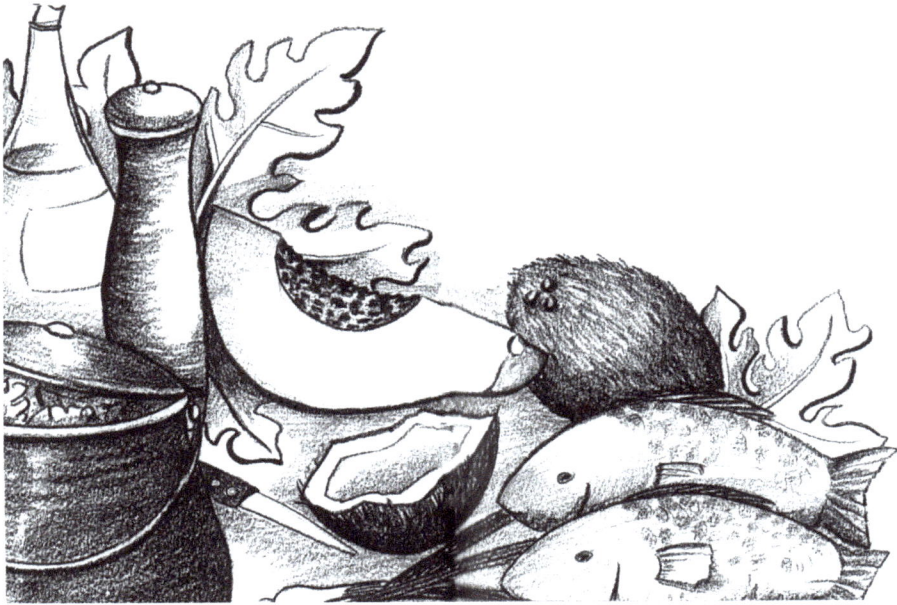

DRESSINGS

EVERYDAY FRENCH

(viniagrette)

1 tbsp French Dijon mustard
salt, pepper
4 tbsp red wine vinegar or cider vinegar
8 tbsp salad oil

- Put mustard in a small bowl, add salt and pepper and mix in vinegar.
- Slowly whisk in oil - a wire whisk is best but a fork or spoon will do.

* It's handy to make this dressing in a screw-top jar. Make any quantity as long as you observe the rule: 1/3rd vinegar, 2/3rds oil - extra mustard can also be added to start with.

VARIATIONS

(to above)

GARLIC VINAIGRETTE

Add 2 or 3 cloves crushed garlic.

HERB VINAIGRETTE

Add a good sprinkling of dried mixed herbs or
dried tarragon or chopped fresh basil or chopped garlic chives.

ITALIAN VINAIGRETTE

Use half salad oil and half olive oil instead of only salad oil.

CREOLE STYLE

2 tsp French Dijon mustard

salt, pepper

2 or 3 spring onions }

1 sprig parsley } *finely chopped together*

2 cloves garlic }

1 tbsp red wine vinegar or cider vinegar

2 tbsp salad oil

(the quantity of vinegar and oil can be varied, keeping the proportions)

- Put mustard, herbs, salt and pepper in small bowl.
- Slowly whisk in vinegar, then oil.

CRUSTACEAN COMPANY

2 heaped tsp French Dijon mustard

2 tbsp salad oil

salt, pepper

juice 1 lime or lemon

parsley -finely chopped

2 or 3 cloves garlic - crushed

- Put mustard in a bowl; whisk in oil drop by drop, as for a mayonnaise.
- Add salt, pepper, lime juice and herbs.

SEED SURPRISE

1½ tbsp ripe papaya seeds
1 heaped tsp French Dijon mustard
½ tsp salt
1 tbsp sugar
1 small onion, chopped
½ cup tarragon vinegar or white vinegar with
sprinkling of dried tarragon
1 cup salad oil

- Put all ingredients, except oil, in blender. Blend well, add oil, blend
  again. Papaya seeds should resemble ground pepper.

* This is a good dressing for rice salad or tossed green salads - especially
if slightly bitter.

WHISKER'S MAYONNAISE

1 egg yolk
2 heaped tsps French Dijon mustard
salad oil - about half a cup
olive oil – about half a cup
salt, pepper
juice of 1 lime or lemon

- Mix mustard into egg yolk in a bowl, then slowly, drop by drop, add oil using a wire whisk, turning always in same direction.
- When mayonnaise is sufficiently mounted add salt, pepper and lime or lemon juice.

* To make a greater quantity, simply keep adding more oil - 1 egg yolk can absorb up to 1 litre of oil!
* If at same time you're making a dish needing 2 egg whites, use 2 egg yolks for a richer mayonnaise.

VARIATIONS (to above)

AIOLI – GARLIC MAYONNAISE

Replace the lime/lemon juice with 4 or 5 cloves of garlic - crushed.

TANGY MAYONNAISE

Increase the quantity of French mustard to 2 tbsp.

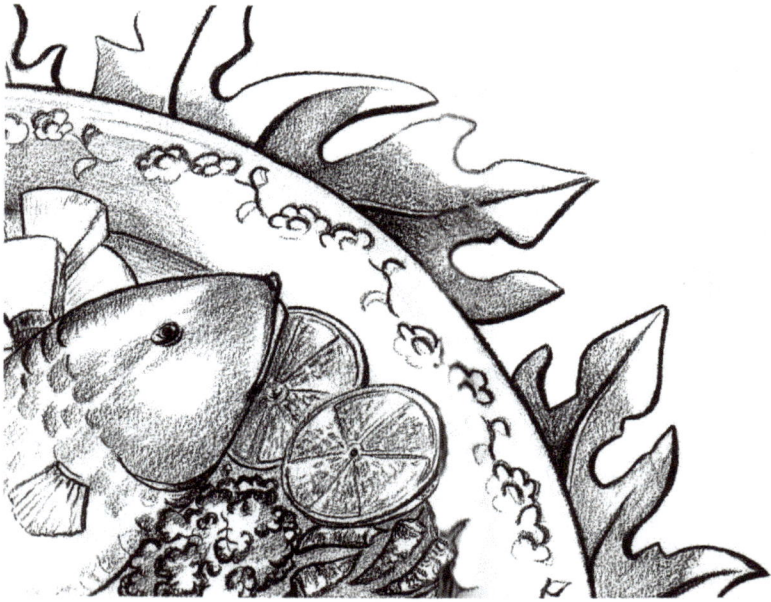

SIDE DISHES for
MEAT or FISH

BUTTERED GREEN

(for 3-4 pers.)

1 medium green papaya
1 tbsp vinegar
salt, pepper
80g (3 oz) butter
parsley - chopped

- Prepare the green papaya and slice thinly.
- Cook in boiling, salted water with vinegar about 10 minutes, till soft. Drain.
- Add butter, parsley and pepper. Serve hot.

* As a variation, add several sticks of celery to the cooking and the juice of half a lime or lemon at the end with the butter.

CROQUETTES

(for 3-4 pers.)

- Prepare same mixture as Indian Ocean entrée/first course without the cheese.
- Roll spoonfuls into balls or tube shapes; dip in breadcrumbs; fry in hot cooking oil.
- Drain on cooking paper.

GREEN PAPAYA PICKLES

(from Geneviève, Noumea)

1 medium green papaya (1 kg)
45 cl water
15 cl white vinegar
3 tbsp salt
50 gr sugar
1 small fresh chilli pepper (de-seeded and finely chopped)
2 tsp mustard seeds
2 tsp coriander seeds

- Peel and de-seed papaya, slice lengthwise then julienne the slices, or grate bigger pieces coarsely.
- Soak papaya in the salt, about 20 minutes, to drain moisture.
- Meanwhile, put water, vinegar, chilli and sugar in a little pan, bring just to the boil so sugar is dissolved.
- Rinse the papaya lightly and, with hands, squeeze out all moisture.
- Put papaya in a bowl, add the mustard and coriander seeds, the sweetened, spiced water and mix well.
- Pack into one large, screw-top jar, or two or three smaller ones. The pickles will be ready after three days.
- Store in fridge. Will keep for weeks.

* Goes well with chicken or fish.

FEARLESS CHUTNEY

(from the yacht, *Fearless*)

(makes about 4 litres, 4 quarts)

1 large papaya - ripe but firm
7 large green mangoes
3 cups white vinegar
1 cup wine vinegar
4 cups sugar
½ cup honey
2 tbsp chili sauce
2 tbsp chili powder (or less depending on personal taste)
1½ tbsp cinnamon
8 cloves
1 tbsp freshly-grated ginger
500g (1 lb) sultanas

- Peel, de-seed and cut fruit into big chunks.
- In a big pan, boil vinegars, sugar and honey.
- Add spices and fruit.
- Boil about 45 minutes.
- Bottle in hot, sterilized jars.

CURRY COMPANY

(for 6 persons)

> 1 small ripe papaya
> 3-4 tbsp vinaigrette or
> 1 small pot (½ cup) of natural unsweetened yoghurt

- Peel, de-seed and dice papaya.
- Put in a small bowl, gently mix in dressing or yoghurt.

* Either way makes a refreshing accompaniment to a hot curry or to a summer salad.

TROPICAL RATATOUILLE

(for 3-4 pers.)

> 1 medium (1 kg / 2-2½ lb) green papaya
> 2 large onions - sliced
> olive oil
> 2 or 3 ripe tomatoes
> 1 small tin (70g / 2½ oz) tomato concentrate
> 1 cup water
> good sprinkling of dried mixed herbs
> salt, pepper

- Prepare green papaya; cut into chunks.
- Heat oil in heavy pot; cook onions till transparent.
- Add chopped tomatoes, tomato concentrate blended with a cup of water, mixed herbs, salt and pepper and papaya. Cover.
- Simmer approx. 20 minutes, stirring now and then.

 * This Tropical Ratatouille goes well with fish grilled, baked, steamed or cooked in a court-bouillon.

ISLAND PUREE

(for 2-3 pers.)

1 medium (1 kg / 2-2½ lb) green papaya
milk
butter
salt, pepper
grated nutmeg or a sprig of thyme

- Prepare as for making mashed potatoes, but use green papaya instead, cooked in salted water. Drain.
- Add milk, a knob of butter, pepper when mashing, and if liked, a dash of nutmeg.

Alternatively, warm milk with a sprig of fresh or dried thyme, before adding to papaya, butter and pepper mixture.

SWEET RIPE

(for 8 persons)

1 small ripe papaya
1 small pineapple
4 spring onions
2 tbsp lemon juice or 1 tbsp lime juice

- Peel and dice fruit.
- Mix with chopped spring onions and lemon or lime juice.
- Serve cooled.

CHILLI RIPE SALSA

(for 6 persons)

1 small ripe papaya, preferably pink
1 small onion or 2 or 3 spring onions
2 tbsp fresh coriander
2 tsp sweet chilli sauce
2 tbsp lime or lemon juice
2 tbsp olive oil
salt & freshly ground pepper

- Peel, de-seed and dice papaya.
- Chop onion and coriander finely.
- Mix all ingredients. Chill to serve.

CRUMBED CHIPS

(for 3-4 pers.)

1 medium (1 kg – 2-2½ lb) green papaya
2 eggs, beaten
1 cup milk
fine breadcrumbs
salt, pepper

- Prepare papaya, cut in half. Cook in boiling, salted water till just soft. Drain.
- Cut into chunky chips.
- Add milk to beaten eggs; dip chips in this, then in breadcrumbs.
- Fry in hot oil. Serve on a hot dish, covered with kitchen paper to drain. Add salt and pepper.
* Do not salt the chips before frying as they will absorb the oil.

SPICEY CHUTNEY from Vanuatu

2kg (4½ lb) firm ripe papaya
juice 1 lime/lemon
125g (4 oz) sugar
3 small chillies, deseeded
1 tsp mustard
2 tbsp fresh ginger, chopped
1 tbsp salt
2 tsp turmeric or curry powder
1 tbsp cornflour mixed with a little water
1 litre (1 quart) vinegar

- Peel papaya, de-seed, cut into small chunks.
- Cover with water and lemon juice; stand for several hours, drain.
- Put in pot just covering with cold water; boil gently 10 minutes then drain again.
- Separately, boil all other ingredients in the vinegar, stirring in papaya when mixture reaches the boil; boil for 20 minutes.
- Bottle into hot, sterilized jars.

MAIN DISHES

FRICASSEE LUNCH

(for 4-5 pers.)

1½ kg (3 lb) green papaya
250g (9 oz) bacon or ham, chopped
1 medium onion, chopped
60g (2 oz) butter
2 cloves garlic
1 tbsp flour
hot water
mixed herbs
pepper,   salt - depending on bacon/ham
parsley

- Prepare papaya, slice like apples.
- Brown bacon and onion gently in frying pan with butter on medium heat.
- Add crushed garlic, then flour to make a roux, stirring till golden.
- Add papaya, stirring; then add hot water, continuing to stir, then mixed herbs, pepper and salt if needed.
- Cover, cook gently 5-10 minutes till papaya is soft.
- Sprinkle with chopped parsley to serve.

HINT OF RAJ

Follow recipe for green papaya curry entrée/first course "Hint of Fiji", increasing quantities if wished and adding more curry powder.

- Add ½-1 cup fresh coconut milk or less tinned coconut cream.
- Serve with plain, boiled rice.
- Garnish with slivers of pickled pink ginger.

HUNTER'S GREEN

(roast of venison tenderised with green papaya)

1 roast of venison
2-3 cloves garlic
cooking oil
2 onions - quartered
1 green papaya
pepper, salt

- Peel & slice garlic, insert into meat all over; dip point of knife into pepper, adding this to garlic holes.
- Prepare papaya, cut into thick slices.
- Heat a little cooking oil in heavy pot, brown meat well; add onions and brown too.
- Add 2 cups water or more, depending on size of roast, stirring browned parts into sauce. Place papaya slices round meat.
- Salt and cook slowly till meat is done, checking regularly to add water if necessary.

* The green papaya not only tenderises the venison, but makes a delicious vegetable accompanying the roast.
* If venison is likely to be especially tough, the day before place papaya slices around meat, leave overnight in fridge and next day prepare as above with the papaya.

PAPAYAUTE

(for 8-10 pers.)

6-8 kg (13-18 lb) green papaya (seeds should be white)
1 dsp (2 tsp) rock salt
100g (3½ oz) lard
300g (11 oz) onions
dry white wine or beer
cracked black pepper
1 tbsp juniper berries
bouquet garni
250g (9 oz) pork rind
pork cuts per person: 1 slice smoked breast
                         1 slice ham
                         1 pork cutlet/chop
                         1 frankfurter
                         2 thick slices garlic salami

    potatoes - steamed

- Prepare papaya and grate like carrots.
- Cover with rock salt for 1 hour then rinse, drain and wring (in a cloth if wished) to draw off liquid.
- Brown sliced onions in lard, then add papaya; moisten with wine or beer; add cracked pepper, juniper berries and bouquet garni.
- In a big, heavy pot lay the pork rind to stop the "papayaute" burning; cover with papaya, onions and wine or beer mixture; lay pork cuts on top.
- Cover; leave to simmer 35-40 minutes.
- Serve with peeled, steamed potatoes.
- * If cooked with white wine, serve white wine to accompany meal; if beer is used, serve beer.

SAM'S SPECIAL

(for 4 pers.)

4 small green papayas (each about the size of an avocado)
meat stuffing :
- 250g (9 oz) cold cooked meat or fresh mincemeat
- 100g (3½ oz) crumbed stale bread without crust, soaked
  in milk or 100g (3½ oz)cooked rice
- 1 medium onion, chopped finely
- 2 or 3 cloves garlic, grated
- 2 tsps sweet chili sauce
- 2 or 3 spring onions, parsley
- mixed herbs - good sprinkling
- salt, pepper
- 1 tbsp ketchup
- 1 egg, slightly beaten
tomato sauce :
- 50g (1½ oz) butter
- 1 or 2 chopped tomato/es
- 3 tbsp ketchup
- fresh or dried thyme
- water
breadcrumbs
grated cheese

- Leave skin on papayas, cut in half, de-seed, cook in boiling, salted water till slightly tender. Drain.
- If using cold meat, mince it.
- Brown chopped onion, stir in cold meat or mincemeat for a few minutes. Add sweet chili sauce.
- In a bowl mix soaked bread or rice, chopped herbs, mixed herbs, meat/onion mix, salt and pepper, ketchup and egg. Stuff each papaya half with this. Arrange in a baking dish.
- Melt butter in small pan, add tomato/es, ketchup, thyme, water, simmer, stirring over a low heat.
- Spoon sauce over each papaya half, sprinkle with breadcrumbs and grated cheese.
- Bake in moderate oven about 20 minutes till papayas are really soft and topping is golden.
- Serve with plain boiled rice.

* Instead of using individual papayas, one medium to large green papaya does equally well - simply cut off the top (keep), scrape out seeds, boil whole till just tender, drain, stuff and put end back, securing it with toothpicks. Serve sliced in rings, dressed with a tomato coulis, accompanied by rice.
* This was one of Sam's regular restaurant dishes.

SUMMER LUNCH

(for 4-5 pers.)

1 medium, firm ripe papaya
1 cold, smoked chicken
3-4 tbsp mayonnaise (or vinaigrette)
black pepper, freshly ground, and salt

- Peel, de-seed and dice most of the papaya, keeping several thin slices for decoration.
- Shred the smoked chicken meat, mix with papaya, mayonnaise, salt and pepper to taste.
- Arrange on serving dish, garnish with thin papaya slices.

* Recipe courtesy of Regent Hotel, Auckland, New Zealand.

TAHITIAN HASH

(for 3-4 pers.)

1 medium green papaya
2 medium onions, chopped
cooking oil
1 tin corned beef
½ cup water
pepper

- Prepare green papaya and grate coarsely.
- Heat oil in frying pan, brown onions; add green papaya, stirring all the time, then corned beef and about ½ cup water.
- Cover, leave to simmer about 5 mins - checking it doesn't dry out.
- Add pepper. Salt only if corned beef is not too salty.

TUNA BOAT

(for 4 pers.)

(an easy dish for lunch during hot weather)

2 small or 1 medium ripe papaya
1 250g (7 oz) tin tuna
250g (9 oz) fresh cottage cheese
freshly-ground black pepper, salt
chopped parsley and 2-3 spring onions
(optional)

- Leave skin on papaya, halve or quarter lengthwise, de-seed.
- Mix drained tuna, cottage cheese and seasonings.
- Fill papaya cavities; serve on individual plates with spoons.

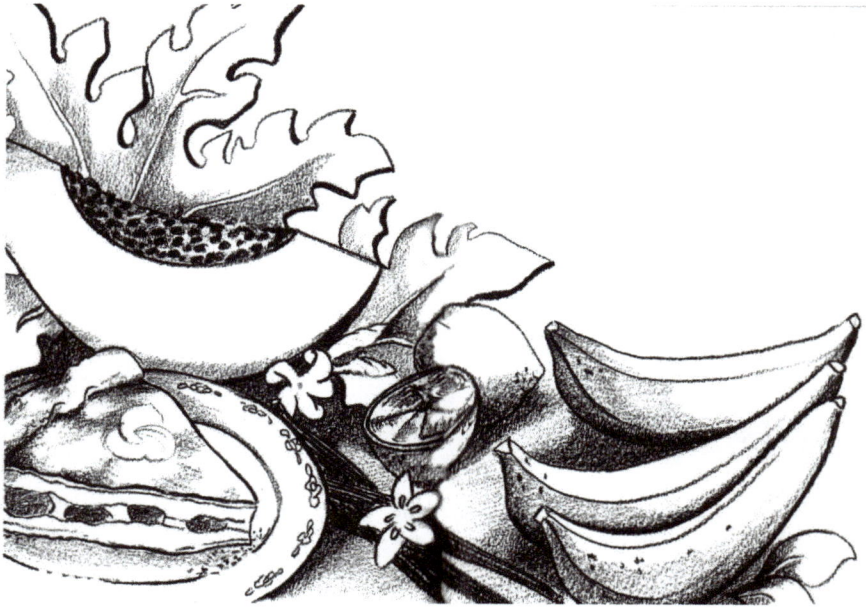

DESSERTS

ANGELS' BREATH

(mousse for 4-6 pers.)

  1 medium, ripe papaya
  juice 1 lime or lemon
  ½ tin unsweetened evaporated milk (chilled); **or**
  250 ml (1 cup) whipping cream
  2 egg whites
  pinch salt
  4 tbsp sugar

- Peel, de-seed and mash or blend papaya; mix in lime or lemon juice.
- In a separate bowl, beat evaporated milk till thick and fluffy or cream till thick.
- In another bowl, beat egg whites with pinch of salt, gradually adding sugar till stiff.
- Gently fold egg whites into cream, then fold in papaya.
- Put in a soufflé-style bowl and set mousse in freezer for an hour or so before serving.

BACCHUS

(for 4-6 pers.)

  1 medium, green papaya
  1 cup red wine
  2 cups water
  1 cup sugar
  1 vanilla bean

- Prepare green papaya; slice like apples and rinse in cold water.
- Put wine, sugar, water and vanilla in a pot, add papaya slices cook gently for 1 hour.
- Serve warm or cold.

BRAZILIAN SIMPLICITY

(per person)

1 generous slice ripe papaya
(unpeeled, de-seeded)
juice of lime or lemon
raw sugar for sprinkling
fresh whipped cream (unsweetened)

- Arrange each slice on individual plates; sprinkle with lemon or lime juice and a little sugar, top with fresh whipped cream.

HONEY HARMONY – Fruit Salad

(for 4-6 pers.)

1 medium, ripe papaya
3 or 4 bananas
3 or 4 passion-fruit
juice 2 limes or lemons
2 tbsp liquid honey
1 tbsp brown rum (optional)

- Peel papaya and bananas - dice and slice.
- Mix in bowl with rest of ingredients.

* The honey adds flavour and a delicate perfume, the rum gives it a little punch!
  They were Sam's special touch to a fruit-salad.
* Alternatively use 3 kiwi fruit and some fresh pineapple instead of or as well as passion-fruit.

CRUMBLE
(for 6 pers.)

1 medium ripe papaya
2 tbsp butter
2 tbsp brown sugar
juice & grated rind of 1 lime or lemon
1 tsp cinnamon
crumble :
6 tbsp flour
3 tbsp brown sugar
3 tbsp butter
100g (3½ oz) chopped walnuts (optional)

- Peel, de-seed and dice the papaya.
- Cook gently for 10 minutes with butter, brown sugar, lime or
  lemon juice and rind and cinnamon.
- Put crumble ingredients in a mixer or rub between fingers to
  obtain crumbs.
- Pour papaya mixture into a buttered ovenproof dish.
- Cover with crumble and cook 20-30 minutes in a moderate oven.
- Serve warm, alone or with whipped cream or vanilla ice-cream.

* This recipe is a family favourite to please all ages.

ENGLISH DELIGHT

(for 4-6 pers.)

> 1 small ripe papaya (500g / 1-1½lb)
> juice 1 lime or lemon
> 3 tbsp custard powder
> ½ litre (2 cups) milk
> 1 tbsp sugar

- Peel, de-seed and mash or blend papaya with lime or lemon juice.
- Make custard: mix custard powder to a smooth paste with a little milk, add sugar to rest of milk - heat till warm, stir in paste and cook several minutes, stirring till custard thickens.
- Blend fruit into hot custard.
- Serve hot or cold.
* For an easier version replace custard with 400ml (1½-2 cups) freshly whipped cream and blend with fruit, lime or lemon juice and a little sugar. Serve chilled.

OVEN RIPE

(for 4-6 persons)

> 1 medium to large ripe papaya
> ½ cup water
> juice 2 limes/lemons
> cinnamon
> 2 tbsp liquid honey or 2 tbsp brown sugar

- Peel and de-seed papaya; cut into 6 or 8 slices lengthwise; arrange in baking dish.
- Pour in water; sprinkle slices with lime juice, honey and cinnamon.
- Bake 15 minutes in moderate oven. Serve hot.

MELBA MEMORY

(for 6-8 pers.)

short pastry for medium-size pie tin or
> 2 cups weetbix
> 1 tbsp brown sugar } mixed together to line tin
> 4 tbsp melted butter

1 medium (1kg / 2-2½lb) ripe papaya
2 tbsp sugar
juice and grated rind of 1 orange   or 2 passion-fruit
1 tbsp butter
1 tbsp cornflour (cornstarch)
2 egg yolks
meringue:
> 2 egg whites
> pinch salt
> 4 tbsp sugar

- Prepare pastry, bake blind a few minutes in moderate oven or line tin with weetbix mixture.
- Prepare papaya, chop roughly; put in pan with orange juice, rind, sugar and butter; stir over low heat till smooth and boiling.
- Blend cornflour with a little water, mix into papaya and continue stirring while mixture thickens.
- Remove from heat; add well-beaten yolks; pour into pastry case.
- Beat egg whites with salt, gradually adding sugar till stiff; spread over papaya.
- Bake in slow to moderate oven about 20 minutes or till golden.
- Cool before serving.

JAM TURNOVERS

puff pastry
papaya jam
1 egg yolk or milk
icing sugar

- Roll out pastry to 1½ cm (¼ inch) thick; with pastry cutter, cut out circles about 8cm (3-4 inches) diameter.
- Put a tablespoonful of jam in centre of each circle; dab edges with cold water, fold in half pressing edges together well.
- Place on greased tray; brush tops with beaten egg yolk or milk; make 2 or 3 incisions in turnovers.
- Bake in moderate oven 20 minutes or till golden.
- Serve slightly warm, sprinkled with icing sugar and accompanied with vanilla ice-cream if desired.

SALUBRIOUS SLICES

(for 8 persons)

1 ripe papaya
1 lime or lemon

- Leave skin on papaya. Cut in half, de-seed then slice lengthwise.
- Arrange attractively on a platter, make several incisions in each slice, squeeze drops of lime or lemon juice on each.

SAM'S FLAMBÉ

(Omelette for 4-6 pers)

1 small just-ripe papaya

3-4 passion-fruit

2 tbsp sugar

4 eggs, separated

pinch salt

1 tsp vanilla essence

2 tbsp butter

1 tbsp cooking oil

3 tbsps brown rum or whisky or brandy

- Peel, de-seed and mash papaya lightly; cut passion-fruit in half, strain off juice; put fruit in pan with 1 tbsp sugar - heat just before adding to omelette.
- Beat egg yolks in a bowl, with 1 tsp water.
- Separately, beat egg whites stiffly with pinch of salt, 1 tbsp sugar and vanilla essence.
- Gently fold yolks into whites.
- Heat butter and oil in a frying pan; pour in mixture, swirling around to cook through evenly; pour heated fruit along middle, fold over both sides to cover middle.
- Slide on to a warmed serving dish; sprinkle with sugar; heat alcohol, pour over omelette and set alight.

• This dessert was Sam's pride and joy.

EASY NEW ZEALAND SORBET

1 medium, ripe papaya
2 passion-fruit
1 lime or lemon
2 tbsp sweetened condensed milk

- Peel and dice papaya, mix with passion-fruit pulp and freeze in small
  quantities (in order to fit into a mixer).
- Thaw fruit mixture slightly. Blend in a mixer, together with the lime
  or lemon juice and condensed milk.
- Refreeze until ready to serve.

SUNSHINE COAST

(per person)

1 generous slice ripe papaya
chopped preserved ginger
fresh whipped cream

- Arrange each slice (with skin on, de-seeded) on individual plates.
- Liberally sprinkle with chopped ginger; serve with cream.

* For an extra touch, add a few drops of sherry to the whipped cream.

TARTIN' UP

(for 6-8 pers.)

350g (12½ oz) short pastry
1 medium (1kg /2-2¼ lb) ripe papaya
80g (3 oz) sugar
80g (3 oz) butter
1 vanilla bean or vanilla essence or cinnamon
fresh cream or ice-cream

- Prepare pastry, roll into a ball, leave in a cool place for 2 hours (or use ready-made pastry).
- Cover pie tin with sugar and butter; melt this over low heat till just blonde.
- Prepare papaya: slice lengthwise in 1-1½cm (¼-½ inch) widths; lay these close together over caramel, like petals.
- Slice vanilla bean in half lengthwise, dab over fruit, or sprinkle with vanilla essence or cinnamon.
- Roll out pastry to size of pie tin; lay pastry over the sliced papaya.
- Cook in moderate oven approx. 25 min. or till golden.
- Turn out tart, pastry-side down, onto oven-proof platter and return to oven to make topside golden.
- Serve warm to cool with fresh cream or vanilla or coconut ice-cream.

THREE SISTERS

(for 8-10 pers.)

1 ripe papaya - yellow or orange flesh
1 ripe pink papaya
1 green papaya
3 limes or lemons
3 tbsp liquid honey
2-3 small pieces vanilla bean or 1 tsp vanilla essence

- Prepare green papaya (rinse off sap, peel & de-seed), quarter, cook in
  boiling water with a little sugar till soft; drain and leave to cool.
- Peel the other papayas, dice along with the cooked green one.
- Mix all with lime or lemon juice, honey and sliced vanilla pieces or
  essence.
- Serve chilled.

TROPICAL CREAM

ripe papaya   } equal quantity of each
ripe bananas   }
juice of 1 lime or lemon
whipped cream (unsweetened) or liquid cream.

- Peel fruit, de-seed papaya.
- Mash with a fork or mix in a blender; add lime or lemon juice, and
  fold in whipped or liquid cream.
- Serve chilled.

TWO Ps SALAD

(for 6-8 pers.)

1 ripe papaya
1 ripe pineapple
1 lime or lemon
2 tbsp liquid honey
vanilla essence or pieces of vanilla
bean
natural yoghurt (unsweetened)

- Peel fruit, de-seed the papaya, dice, mix with lime or lemon juice, honey and vanilla; chill.
- Serve with natural yoghurt to accompany.

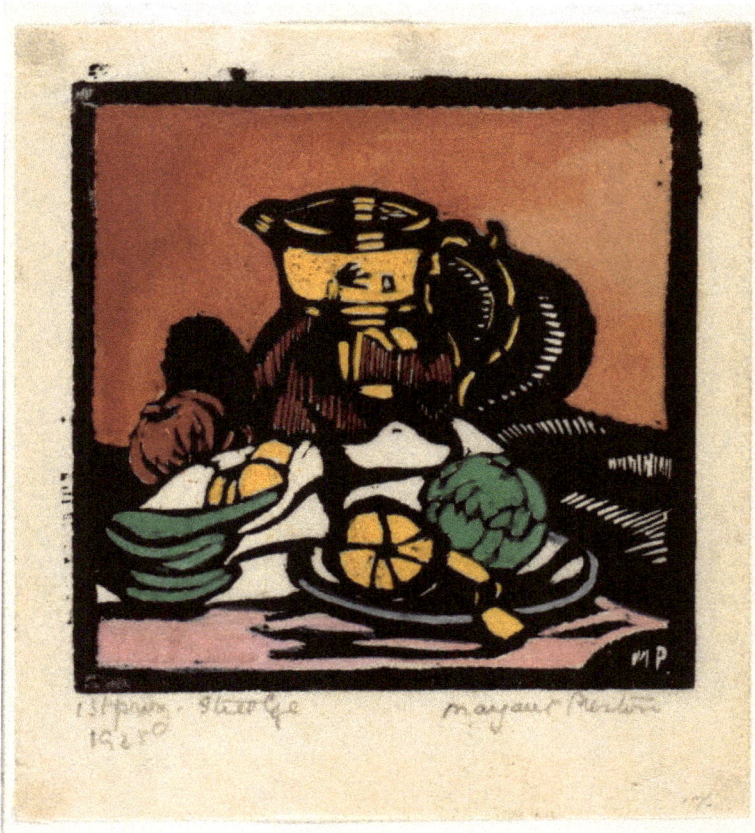

COFFEE COMPANY

CRYSTAL GREEN

1 medium (1 kg / 2-2½ lb) green papaya
peel of 1 lime or lemon
1 kg (2¼ lb) sugar
½ litre (2 cups) water

- Prepare green papaya, slice into 8 lengthwise.
- Peel lime or lemon; add this peel to papaya, sugar and water; cook about 3/4 hour till water is reduced to a thick syrup and papaya is soft. Leave to cool.
- Put papaya and syrup in an airtight jar to keep. Or remove papaya from syrup, toss pieces in castor sugar, put on a rack to dry in the sun or air for one day; keep in a jar.

* This is handy to serve with coffee when there's no dessert.

PAPAYA MUFFINS

(makes 12)

¼ cup oil
½ cup liquid honey
½ cup natural yoghurt
1 egg
1 cup chopped ripe papaya
grated rind of 1 lemon or orange
several pieces of vanilla bean or ½ tsp vanilla essence
2 cups self-raising flour or
   2 cups plain flour and 3 tsps baking powder (sifted)
150ml (2/3 cup) milk
1 tsp bicarbonate of soda

- Preheat oven to moderately hot (375ºF) and butter the muffin tin or silicon moulds.
- Thoroughly combine all ingredients except flour, milk and bicarb.soda. Then fold these in alternatively.
- Pour into muffin tin or moulds, filling each compartment to the top; bake 15-20 minutes. The muffins are ready when they're firm to touch and move slightly away from the edge of the tin.
- Leave in tin for five minutes, before turning out on to a rack to cool.

4 O'CLOCK

300g (11 oz) firm, ripe papaya
grated rind of 2 lemons
250g (10 oz) self-raising flour
125g (4½ oz) butter
½ tsp vanilla essence
1 egg
1dl (½ cup) milk
1 tsp cinnamon
125g (4½ oz) sugar plus 1 tbsp sugar

- Pre-heat the oven to moderate temperature.
- Peel, de-seed and slice papaya thinly, as for apples. Add lemon rind.
- Sieve flour.
- Cream butter and sugar; when fluffy add vanilla essence, a little flour, the egg, then flour and milk alternatively.
- Pour half this mixture into a buttered, loaf tin.
- Neatly lay half the papaya; sprinkle with half cinnamon and sugar.
- Cover with other half of cake mixture, then papaya, cinnamon and sugar.
- Cook 35-45 minutes in a moderate oven. Test if cooked with a fork. Serve cold.

OTHER BOOKS IN THE
SYDNEY-PARIS LINK SERIES:

The Thorn in the Flesh
Paul Wenz
Their Father's Land
Paul Wenz
Australasian Artists at the French Salons
Tom Thompson
Village to Village
Alister Kershaw
Journal of a Political Exile in Australia
Leon Ducharme
Notes of a Convict of 1838
Xavier Prieur
Diary of a New Chum
Paul Wenz
Food for Friends
Babette Hayes
Australian Painters at Etaples
Jean-Claude Lesage
One Rose in Bali
Hilary Roots
Reciprocity: A Celebration on the Life of
Jean-Paul Delamotte

www.ingramcontent.com/pod-product-compliance
Lightning Source LLC
LaVergne TN
LVHW010316070426
835513LV00021B/2406